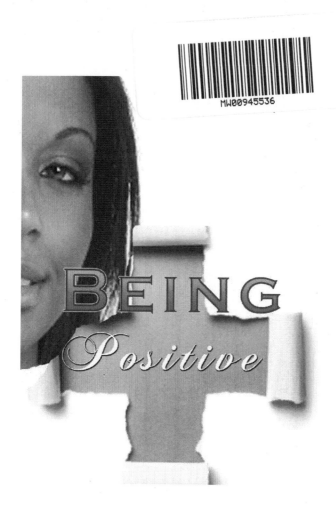

# BEING
## *Positive*

# BY KIMBERLIN DENNIS

*Kimberlin Dennis*
# BEING POSITIVE

For many people "Being Positive" with HIV/AIDS is impossible but Kimberlin Dennis has managed to use her diagnosis as an opportunity to minister and uplift others.

Through testimony, "Being Positive" will answer the questions that many people are afraid to ask. Questions Like:

"How do people contract HIV?"
"Can you live a normal life after you have been diagnosed?
"What are the early symptoms?"

"Being Positive" gives you the one-on-one encounter of Kimberlin's experience after she received a positive HIV test result. Twenty years later, Kimberlin is an author, motivational speaker & the founder of Ministry of Hope, Inc.

**In Memory of**

My biggest cheerleader and my number one supporter, my mother Mrs. Barbara Jean Battle

September 12, 1943 – January 21, 2009

"You don't have to be infected to be affected by HIV/AIDS!"

## Dedication

This book is dedicated to my husband Darryl Edward Dennis. Sputnik, before you left, you told me that I would be okay, and that you knew I could go on living with this disease. Look at me now...two decades later, and I am okay.

This is not just my story; it is OUR story.

To my cousin and the Ministry of Hope co-founder Jacqueline Marie Hatten for her tireless work and energy that she gave to the Ministry of Hope, and believing in me, knowing that the book would get done and would be a blessing to so many people. She helped start the ministry with me; she believed in my dream that God wanted this to continue. Rest in peace cousin, I still hear you talking to me, every time I need you.

## Table of Contents

## Foreword

It has truly been my honor and privilege to be Kimberlin Dennis's physician for the past 22 years. In this book, she shares --- honestly and poignantly --- the story of her marriage to Darryl, his rapid and untimely death from AIDS, and the remarkable journey she has traveled since first learning in 1994 of her own HIV infection. The changes have been extraordinary. During that time, HIV infection has evolved from a near-uniformly fatal infection to a manageable chronic infection, at least in those parts of the world and in those populations who have access to modern health care and medications. In parallel, Kim has evolved from a bewildered and nearly overwhelmed young widow to a confident, open, well-informed, and eloquent representative and educator on the subject of living with HIV infection.

Kim recognized a long time ago that regardless of what modern medicine and technology could offer her, she could not accept, learn, survive, and flourish without acknowledgment and acceptance of a High Power. Her life is a witness to that power. Her example has taught me so much --- about the things that patients and their doctors need to hear and share as they work together to sustain health, and about the awesome power of hope.

David Hutt, MD

February 2016

*Kimberlin Dennis*
# BEING POSITIVE

## Introduction

As a little girl, I was sick a lot. My mother was constantly in the hospital with me. In fact, I think I had pneumonia nine times when I was young. As the middle sibling of three sisters, I am not sure if I suffered from the middle child syndrome or not. My father was strict but my mother disciplined us the most; therefore, having both parents in the house was a blessing and a curse. We had a lot of fun growing up but when we did something wrong we suffered the consequences.

My mother made it easy for my sisters and me to talk to her about anything. We used to have girl talk about everything. Although they did not always share with me, I always shared my things with my sisters. It did not matter if it was my favorite item or something new, I allowed them to wear or utilize them before I did. I realized at an early age that I am a giver and I enjoy giving. I always stayed to myself; however, my two sisters had their friends. Many people in school did not know we were sisters until one of them told.

I attended Cleveland Public Schools and worked in the school office; I liked to help the teachers. I wanted to be a school- teacher when I grew up. I taught a 12th grade workshop for my summer school job, and I was only in the 10th grade at the time. The teacher died and there was only a few weeks left of summer school. Instead of bringing in a new teacher to finish, they let me finish out the last few weeks of summer school, since I already knew the lessons. The students needed a good grade in order to graduate. I was firm and gave each student the grade they had earned. A couple of students was troublemakers and did not like the grade they earned so they would smoke in the class and make noise. They went as far as throwing a smoke bomb into the class and we all had to go outside, but everyone was fine. Most of the students in class were good because they wanted to graduate. That experience discouraged me; I did not want to be a teacher anymore.

After I graduated from high school, I went to Tri-C College to get a degree in Business Education. After being in college for two years, I was hired at the State of Ohio building located in downtown Cleveland in 1982; however, I never finished my college degree.

## BEING POSITIVE

In 1983, I was still living with my parents. My oldest sister would be gone with her friends and boy did she have a lot; my youngest sister would be gone too, but she would be somewhere with a boy. She had girlfriends too, but she liked one boy whom she spent a lot of time with. I had friends, but I stayed to myself.

One day I was looking out my bedroom window at the street in front of our house. As I was looking out the window, a motorcycle pulled up. I could hear my parents talking to the man on the bike. My mother called me down to the porch and asked me if I knew who he was and I said no. I knew his uncle and mother, but I really did not know him.

Our families grew up together. My father's side of the family was so big, we had to have a family reunion because a lot of us first cousins were in school together and we did not know we were related. A few of us, including me, were dating one of our cousins and did not know it until our first reunion. We were dating for only one week at the time and it is a good thing nothing happened. We found out we were not the only ones either, so we still have family reunions today for that reason. We would have fundraisers to raise money to have the family reunions. It had to be about the fourth or fifth one we were having, so all of the first cousins decided to give our first fundraiser to help towards the reunion. We decided to host a cabaret and we called ourselves the "Second Generation."

We had our cabaret at Camelot Hall, where I met Darryl. He saw me setting up behind the bar and he kept asking me to dance. I was busy, so I kept pushing him away. Finally, I went to dance with him and while we were dancing, he asked me to be his girlfriend and I said "I don't know." Well, my oldest sister was fast and quick and she told me that I had until midnight the next day to make up my mind or else Darryl was going to be her man. She told me she was being nice because I was her sister, otherwise she would have had him already and thought nothing of it. I waited until June 12, 1991 at 11:59 p.m. to tell Darryl 'yes, I would be his girlfriend'.

We had fun together. We would go out to eat, dance, concerts, family functions, laugh and have a good time. I loved to see Darryl laugh. He had the prettiest smile and his teeth were so white. As dark as he was, he would light up the place. When Darryl smiled it made me smile more; we were happy and in love. We dated for three years. One day, Darryl and I were at his mother's house, where he lived. While we were there, Darryl got down on one knee and asked me to marry him. I laughed at him until I realized he was serious. He did not have a ring so I thought he was playing around; however, I said yes.

We set the wedding date for August 22, 1987. My oldest sister was so happy; she tried to run things her way. She was going to be my bridesmaid, but she did not like the colors I picked out, gray and fuchsia. She said she was going to wear what she wanted as well as the color she wanted, and we fought about it.

On December 27, 1986 my oldest sister, Robin was murdered two days after Christmas.

She was so happy about Darryl and me getting married. The death of my sister left me unsettled. We had to go to the trial from January of 1987 to June of 1987, and our wedding was set for August 22, 1987. We had to make some changes and try to get things done in two months, but it was one thing after another. The day of the wedding the bridesmaids did not have their dresses to wear, the woman that was making all the dresses including my dress was a friend of my mother-in-law.

The girlfriend of Darryl's best man had bought a wedding dress just in case she got married. It was a brand new dress and she gave me her dress to wear, thank God it fit. Darryl kept calling me to find out what was taking us so long to get to the church because the people at the church were getting restless. Darryl said just come to the church, he was not marrying a dress he was marrying me and he did not care what I had on. My father and I went to the church while the bridesmaids were at my house all made-up but they had no dresses.

Darryl had picked out seven girls to stand with his groomsmen. My youngest sister had just had her second son on August 19, 1987, so she could not be my bridesmaid either and my oldest sister had died. My youngest sister was released from the hospital the day of my wedding. She came to the wedding, but could not go to the reception, so I asked my sister-in-law if she would be my bridesmaid and she said yes. My mother-in-law went over to the woman's house, picked up all the dresses and brought them to the church.

All I know is that it was a Cinderella wedding. I was in someone else's dress, but I walked down the aisle in my own dress. I had seven bridesmaids with no dresses; they came to the church in their robes. However, by the time they showed up their dresses were coming out of the trunk of the car and all seven bridesmaids had on their dresses. My husband's cousin was a tailor and she sewed the dresses on the girls so fast, it had to be God working. The wedding was almost four hours late but everyone stayed. We got married and had the reception at Camelot Hall. We went to Hawaii for our honeymoon for 7 days.

When we got back, Darryl and I lived with my parents until we moved into our new house on May 21, 1988. We wanted a house we could enjoy and have kids. We traveled and enjoyed life before we were ready to have kids.

Darryl loved kids so we had our niece and nephews all the time. My youngest sister had four boys and my sister-in-law had two boys and one girl. My husband's nickname was Sputnik, but people called him Spud. His mother gave him that nickname, because he was born the year the rocket Sputnik went up into space. Our niece and nephews loved them some Uncle Spud. Darryl loved basketball and he would take them to his games. He would spend a lot of time with them just having fun either playing video games, sports, playing in the snow, in the yard, or just going for a ride somewhere. Darryl loved to drive and I enjoyed the rides.

I was 26 years old when we got married and Darryl was 29 years old. We had a dog-named Kit. It was Darryl's baby before we got married and when we bought our house, she came to live with us. My parents also had a dog and his name was Shadow. He was an all-black Doberman and Kit was an all-red Doberman.

My parents had three girls, but we loved to watch sports with our dad and I still do to this day. My husband and I loved to watch sports together as well. I also like to watch the news because my grandmother, on my father's side, used to make us be quiet when the news was on and we had to watch it with her. So today, I still watch the news a lot.

## Chapter One

In 1994, Darryl started to develop bumps on the back of his hands. We did not know what they were, but they kept coming up all over his body. We went to the doctor and they ran every test they could. All of the tests came back with good results. One of the tests Darryl had to have was a bone marrow test. They had to stick a long needle into his spine. He did not like needles and it hurt me just to see him try to keep still and bear the pain of that test. That one also came back good and he did not have Tuberculosis.

In 1991, I got pregnant; Darryl and I were ecstatic because we wanted children so bad. I was a couple of months pregnant and I was over at my parents' house laying on the couch with morning sickness. I had a doctor's appointment the next day; my mother was a nurse's aide at St. Luke's Hospital at the time. She told me that everything was going to be all right.

I went to the doctor out on 185th and Lakeshore and my parents lived on Dove off 116th Street. My husband, Darryl, was at work. When I went in for the appointment with Dr. Brzozowski, my OB/GYN, he did an ultrasound and told me that the baby was growing outside the placenta and that I was going to have a miscarriage. It was not normal and the baby would be deformed or would not make it. It was not normal for a baby to be growing outside the placenta. He gave me some pills that would cause me to miscarry.

I cried all the way back to my parents' house. I was on the 90 West Freeway driving fast and crying blaming my mother because she said everything was going to be all right and for me not to worry. The day before when I was lying on the couch, I felt like something was wrong. I knew it was not my mother's fault, but I was angry with her and God. I cried so hard I really could have killed myself and hit someone on the freeway as fast as I was going; but God let me make it home safely.

Darryl came home from work and got me and we went home to our house. Darryl got a call saying his great grandmother had died and he had to go down to Atlanta for the funeral. I had never met his great grandmother, but I heard a lot about her and talked to her on the phone once. I could not go because I had to take the pills to abort the baby. I stayed home and Darryl drove with his family down to Atlanta for the funeral. He did not want to leave me at home, but I could not go.

Darryl was so worried he called home every chance he had. I do not think cellphones were out then, if so, we did not have one yet. The day Darryl came back home is when I had the miscarriage. The pain was so strong, I went to the bathroom and it came out. I cried and called the doctor. Darryl had just got home and had to take me to the doctor; they cleaned me out and sent me back home.

It was not long after that I was pregnant again. I knew I was, so I thought the morning sickness was normal. I did not tell anyone at work, just Darryl's family and myself knew. We wanted to make sure this time before we told everybody else.

I rode the bus to work in the morning and Darryl would pick me up when I got off. We only had the one car and Darryl had to be at work at 6:00 a.m. and I had to be at work at 8:00 a.m. Darryl got off work at 3:00 p.m. and I got off at 4:45 p.m. That day I was on the seven bus going to work downtown at the State Building. I did not feel good at all, but I knew I was pregnant so I thought it was morning sickness. One morning as I walked through the Terminal Tower to get to work, my cousin spoke to me as she was getting off the rapid. I was in a daze and I do not remember me responding. I would get to work early, so I could eat breakfast before 8:00 a.m. at my desk.

I was sitting at my desk and I still did not feel good. All of a sudden, my head hit the desk, it was cold and it felt good. People were walking by looking, but I could not move. I told them I was pregnant so my boss and co-workers called the State Building nurse's office and they sent a wheelchair up to the seventh floor to get me.

I went and laid on the bed in the nurse's office. I told her I was pregnant and maybe I was just having morning sickness. I had eaten an orange and that is all I had. The more I lay there the worse I got, so the nurse called my mother to come and get me.

When I got into the Arrow star van, I blacked out while I was laying on the back seat and my mother took me to her house. When we got there, I blacked out again while getting out the van. Going into the house, my father and sister were home playing with a learning game that had just come in the mail. I went to lie on the couch; they knew I was pregnant and thought I was having morning sickness too. I kept blacking out, so my sister was putting cold wet rags on me in all the creases over my body, between my legs, arms, neck, forehead, and it felt good.

I had to go to the bathroom and it was 15 steps up the flight of stairs. My father, mother and sister tried to help me to the bathroom and on the way up, I blacked out again. When I got into the bathroom while sitting on the toilet, I blacked out again. I could hear them screaming my name, my mother said, "Let's take her to the hospital."

My parents worked at St. Luke's and were arguing about which hospital they should take me. My father said not St. Luke's because everyone knew each other and everyone's business. My mother said, "So what?" She just wanted to get me to a hospital.

My sister was still pouring cold water on me with wet rags. She poured all of the cold water that was in the refrigerator into a bucket, put the rags in it, and brought it with us in the van. My parents were still arguing about which hospital to take me. Darryl was at work; we did not even think to call him.

They took me to Dr. Brzozowski's office in Beachwood Place. When I got there I went into shock, they called the ambulance to come and get me. At that moment, Darryl walked in the doctor's office. He said he felt something was wrong; he left work and came to the doctor's office. No one called him to tell him where we were or what happened. He said God led him there. Darryl got in the front seat of the ambulance with me in the back. My mother drove our car and my father drove the van with my sister, and they followed the ambulance to University Hospital ER.

On the way to the hospital, the workers asked me if I could lift up so they could take my pants off. They were trying to avoid cutting them off to put me into a body bag stabilizer, so I lifted up my bottom just enough so they could slide my pants off and at that moment I blacked out again in the ambulance. Darryl was in the front and he opened the window to look in the back where I was and they kept shutting it. I could hear the window shutting back and forth. I kept blacking in and out and they were saying "Code Blue."

When I got in the hospital, they put me on a table. They could not find a place to put the IV in so it had to go into my big toe. I kept telling them to hurry up. My jaws were flapping, my body was shaking and I was going into shock. I remember going to sleep and praying to God. I knew that I could not breathe and I could see myself lying on the emergency room table. I had an out-of-body experience and I kept trying to tell the doctors that I could not breathe. I realized that they could not hear me. I was praying to God for help, I was in a peaceful tunnel and I could see a bright light at the end. I knew I did not want to go there. I knew I had died.

When I woke up, I saw my sister's husband at my bedside. When I opened my eyes, I scared him as he thought I was dead. I had tubes all in me, machines were going and a tube was down my throat. My sister's husband ran out the room, down the hall and when he got to the elevator, my uncle (who was a pastor) was getting off. My uncle was coming to pray for me. He brought my brother-in law-back to my room and my uncle held my left hand and my sister's husband held my right hand; my uncle said a prayer for me, then they left. I kept looking around to see where I was, because I knew I had died. I could not talk because the tubes were in my mouth.

The next day my mother, grandmother, and husband came to see me. My mother was cleaning me up because blood was all over me, from head to toe. I could see the bloody water, back then you had to wash up in a silver washbowl and my mother kept changing the water. I kept asking her where all that blood was coming from and my mother would say,

"Girl be quiet and let me clean you up." Darryl was looking in through the door and my grandmother was watching my mother wash me. I asked where my jewelry was. I wore a ring on every finger, two-necklaces, an ankle bracelet, a watch and a bracelet. My mother showed me a big plastic bag and all of my jewelry was in it including my wedding ring.

I still wanted someone to tell me what had happened. My grandmother said I had an ectopic pregnancy and died, they gave me two quarts of blood to save my life. My grandmother was not happy because she was a Jehovah Witness so she did not agree with the process. I was just glad to be alive and I did not care whose blood it was. The doctors did not have time to ask anyone for permission because it was a matter of life and death.

When they opened me up, they said blood splattered all over the walls and ceiling in the emergency room. I had lost a lot of blood that was when I could not breathe.

The doctors took my husband and mother into a room; they said we have good and bad news. They told them the bad news first, that I had died and that they had to give me two quarts of blood to save me. My mother passed out and they had to give her some smelling salt to wake her up. Then they told her and my husband the good news that I was alive and was going to be ok. My sister really saved my life, by putting the cold rags on me; it was freezing the blood and stopping it from spreading to my organs, thank you God.

My father did not want me to leave the hospital until I had an HIV test. My father and grandmother were mad about the blood transfusion, but I was just glad to be alive. The hospital tested me for HIV/AIDS and my results came back negative. I had to go back three months later to be re-tested again and it was negative again.

**Chapter Two**

At this point, Darryl had taken every test there was to take; the doctors were trying to figure out what was wrong. His doctor had referred him to Dr. Hutt around March 1, 1994. I remember Darryl and me going to see Dr. Hutt for the first time at University Hospital.

We were in a waiting room; Dr. Hutt walked in. He examined Darryl and looked over Darryl's file. Dr. Hutt saw all of the tests Darryl had taken including the bone marrow test. Dr. Hutt said he would like to do one more test on Darryl, an HIV test. Darryl said ok, because we both wanted to know what was wrong. Darryl wanted the doctors to find out what was wrong so they could treat the problem and make him well again. Dr. Hutt asked Darryl if he had any questions. Darryl said, "What are all these sores that are all over my body." and Dr. Hutt said they looked like lesions. Darryl asked if he could give him something to make them go away. Dr. Hutt said, "Go get your blood work done and after you take the HIV test come back in two weeks to see me." and he said to get some Benadryl for the itching. He gave Darryl a prescription for the pain. We left the hospital.

On the way back home, it was so quiet in the car you could hear a pen drop. I was praying in my mind to God, "Lord what is wrong with my husband, please let him get well." I do not think either of us thought about the HIV test at that moment because every test Darryl had taken came back good. We really thought the HIV test was going to come back good as well. We had heard about HIV/AIDS from the TV on the news and when Magic

Johnson told the world, he had it in 1991. The little we knew about HIV/AIDS was it did not fit our lifestyle. We had to wait two weeks before the results came back. Darryl was so sick; he was trying to get through one day at a time. The days were getting hard to get through most of the time. In the two-week wait, we talked about what if the test shows that he was HIV positive. At the same time, we felt it was not HIV, because we went back and forth over our life and HIV just did not suit our lifestyle. The lifestyle for HIV/AIDS in 1994 was called a "Gay White man's disease" (White men who were having sex with men). Darryl was not gay nor white and neither was I, so how could this be.

On March 21, 1994, my father's mother was rushed to St Luke's Hospital. The family was going to see her. After being in a coma for a week, my aunt who lived with my grandmother died. It was my father's baby sister, the youngest out of 12 kids. On the same day, Darryl got his results back.

Dr. Hutt told Darryl he was positive and that he only had three months to live. Dr. Hutt told him to do whatever he wanted to within three months. Darryl was so sick; he could not travel or even try to enjoy his last days. So much was going on at that time. I remember the ride back home with Darryl; all he could do was cry. He was so worried about my family and myself. He told me to go over to my parents' house to be with my family.

I had taken a HIV test that same day Darryl was diagnosed. I drove him home; I could see the two of us leaving Dr. Hutt's office for the first time quiet and still not knowing what to say. I truly believe that we both were having our moment with God. I know I was talking and praying to God, and I know Darryl was too, even in the stillness and quietness in the car ride home. I dropped him off at the door of our house and I went over to my parent's house. I cried all the way over there, I did not know what to do. I knew Darryl was going in the house to cry and to call his mother and sister to tell them what his results were.

I got over to my parents' house and my father got in the car with me. My mother drove her Arrow Star Van and my father's brother rode with my mother. We went over to my grandmother and aunt's house to be with the family while they arranged for my aunt's funeral. On the way over there, I just cried uncontrollably. My father thought all my tears were for my aunt, and for my grandmother, who was still in the hospital. My tears were for them too, but they were also for the devastating news about Darryl being told he had AIDS and that he did not have long to live. I told my father about Darryl's diagnosis in the car when we were driving over to the house where all my family was.

When I told my dad, all he could do was drop his head. He asked how Darryl was doing. I told him I did not know, but it is not good. We did not talk in the car on the way home. I told my dad I had taken the HIV test again before I left the hospital and in two weeks, I would know where I stood. My dad knew I had a lot on me then. I felt like I was in a daze, I was so quiet; all I could do was cry. I left and my dad said he would ride back home with my mother.

Another aunt asked me to give her a ride home; she lived a couple of streets from where my grandmother and aunt lived, her mother and sister. I took her home; my aunt was a Jehovah Witness. I did not say a word the whole time she was in my car. When I pulled up in her driveway, she looked at me and said, "Can I say something?" I said, "Yes, go right ahead." She said, "I don't know what you are going through right now. I know Darryl is sick and you have been taking care of him, and I know you have a lot more on your shoulders than any of us right now." She told me to promise her that I would give all my problems to Jehovah God, that I would put them in his hands and leave them there, to trust Jehovah God and believe He will take care of it all. I cried and said, "Ok, I will." She got out the car and I left.

I cried all the way home, because no one knew that Darryl had just been told he had AIDS, but my father and myself. I did not want to tell my mother, because I did not think she could handle it. My father told my mother, because he needed her. My mother was stronger than I thought she would be.

The day we buried my aunt, I had to leave the church early and go to Dr. Hutt's office on Park Place to get my results. I had to meet Darryl there because he had an appointment with Dr. Hutt as well. Darryl's mother and sister drove him to Dr. Hutt's office. I walked in and saw Darryl; he was lying on the table waiting for his examination. Dr. Hutt came in and asked me to come with him to his office. I followed him and I knew then I was HIV positive too. I could see it on Dr. Hutt's face. When I sat down in the chair in his office I said, "I'm HIV positive." and he said, "Yes you are." I asked him how long I had to live. He said that I was just positive for HIV and not AIDS. There was no time limit on my life like Darryl's.

Dr. Hutt answered all my questions. He asked me if I wanted him to be my doctor too and I said yes. He told me he wanted to see me for an appointment and that he felt it was best. I told Darryl that I was HIV positive and that he was the one who infected me. I asked Dr. Hutt about the ectopic pregnancy. I asked Dr. Hutt if he could tell Darryl for me, because

I could not. He asked my sister and mother-in-law to step out the room for a moment, but I said to let them stay. I wanted them to hear it too. Dr. Hutt told Darryl that I was HIV positive and that he was the one who infected me. Darryl told Dr. Hutt to promise him that he would take good care of me. Dr. Hutt said, "No, my job is to take good care of you both." I left and went back to my parents' house and Darryl left and went with his mother and sister.

My grandmother had died on the last Sunday in March 1994, which was Easter Sunday. When my aunt died, Darryl got his results. When my grandmother died, I got my results a day before; it was a Saturday morning. I spent a lot of time talking and praying to God, and so did Darryl. He read the bible so fast word for word. He prayed and talked to God every second of the day. Darryl's sister and I would read the bible to Darryl when he could not read on his own, jaundice had now set in and it was hard for him to read.

Kimberlin Dennis

# BEING POSITIVE

## Chapter Three

Before meeting me, Darryl dated a girl in high school who he later found out was an IV drug user. They broke up and he moved back home with his mother. When we met, Darryl told me about her and that when he found out about her drug use he left her and moved back home; he never would have thought her drug behavior would have an effect on our lives. She got HIV from IV drug use, gave it to Darryl through unprotected sex. He was so hurt that she did not tell him, knowing we were getting married. She knew before we got married, because she left Cleveland and moved to California.

Darryl and I did not drink we just smoked marijuana. I never did any hard drugs, but I also learned to never, say never. I thank God every day of my life and I pray that I still do not smoke. Dr. Hutt told me it was ok for me to continue smoking marijuana. It was helping me in a lot of ways, appetite, stomach pain and nausea. I kept on smoking it until one day it no longer helped. I was not eating but smoking all day from the time I got up, to the time I went to bed.  In January of 2005, I decided to stop smoking. I do not miss it and thank God, I can manage my health without it.

Darryl and I dated for three years before we got married.  We were married seven years when we were diagnosed.  Darryl was 36 years old and I was 33 years old.

Darryl worked at Basic Aluminum; he would never take off from work even when he was sick.   When  I  met  him  he  had  a motorcycle, but he would drive my car to work or  ride  the  bus.   They  made  parts  for  Ford

Motor Co., so it would be hot in there, 10 to 20 degrees hotter than outside. Darryl worked hard and only took off on holidays.

When Darryl got sick, he had many days accumulated. Darryl thought that this would be a good time for him to take a sick leave and then go back to work. He thought a week or two would be enough rest. The lesions began to spread all over him from head to toe. At some point, he was too sick to return to work. He began to get weak and could no longer play basketball. Not being able to work or play really hurt him. His health was failing and the doctor's still did not know what was wrong. Darryl and I were living a wonderful life. We had a beautiful house, good jobs and a nice car and truck. We went from being happy to now living a secret, the secret we could not tell.

The stigma of HIV/AIDS was and still is so strong. People treat you as if you are contagious; look at you as if you are dirty, nasty, and filthy. The first thing a person asks when they find out you are HIV Positive is, "How did you get it?" People still think if you touch, or kiss someone you can get it, and that is not true. People treat you as if you have a plague. They do not want to hug you or be near you. All a person wants is to be loved. Darryl did not want people to know he was dying of AIDS because he did not want to be stigmatized as something he was not. Remember, at that time, HIV/AIDS was considered a gay white man's disease. What people do not understand is that HIV does not discriminate, it does not care what your sexual preference is, and it does not care what age or race you are.

Darryl could not believe he was dying of AIDS, being a 36-year-old black, straight man. How could it happen to us? He was hurt and felt like his life was being taken from him too soon. He did not want his family and friends to know because he did not want to answer all the questions that people wanted to know: "How did you get it? Are you gay? This *is* a gay man's disease!" He also did not want to be scrutinized and be told: "Don't touch me, or come near me, or eat at my house, or off of my dishes." Darryl just did not want people to feel uncomfortable around him. Everywhere he went; people would stare at him because of his lesions, and ask, "What is that?" or "How did that happen?"

I never got lesions and I would put Aloe Vera on Darryl to help ease the itching and scratching. I prayed to God, for help. Before she was murdered, my sister Robin purchased an Aloe Vera plant and when we bought our new house; my mother let me have it. My sister told me it was a medicine plant. I told her, "Yeah, right." but when I prayed to God for help with Darryl, I looked at that plant in the window and I asked Darryl if I could put it on his skin. He said yes, and it helped a lot; his skin was clearing up. I would put it all over from head to toe. It cooled his skin down and stopped the itching. His hair and skin was smooth. The plant was big and full when I first started to use it, then it got thin. I had to buy another one. I also bought Aloe Vera juice for him to drink, so it could work from the inside out, and the plant could work from the outside in.

Darryl had reached the point where he did not want to go anywhere. He did not want people coming over to our house to visit. He knew they just wanted to see him and talk about him, or how he was looking. He was about 6 feet 4 inches tall and weighed 165 plus pounds; he had gone down to 90 pounds. I also lost weight I went from 145 to 90 pounds, results of HIV/AIDS.

*Kimberlin Dennis*
# BEING POSITIVE

## Chapter Four

On January 21, 1994, Darryl's mother gave him a birthday party fundraiser to help pay for some of the medical bills. He came to the party but he was so sick he had to leave early. He had lost a lot of weight and the lesions were still all over his body. He came because it was his birthday.

We did not find out until two months later in March 1994 what was wrong, and that was when he was diagnosed with AIDS. Darryl was staying with his mother so his grandmother and aunt could watch him while his mother, sister and I worked. I would leave our home, go to work then go over to my mother-in-law's house to spend time with Darryl. It was hard for me to go back and forth, and I was sick as well. He had gotten to the point where he would wait for me to come to clean him up and try to get him to eat something. His appetite was gone; he felt bad about not being able to do for himself.

Bills were getting behind at our house; my income was the only one coming in. Darryl and I had a black 1989 Oldsmobile. Once it was paid off, Darryl purchased a 1993 Chevy Blazer truck. It was black, trimmed in red going down the side; it was two-toned. We had a new truck that had a note to pay each month and he was not working, just me. It had gotten hard for me to do for him and myself, so he called me at work and said he wanted to come back home. My mother-in-law did not want me to bring him home, so he stayed at his mother's house for about six months from January 1994 to July 1, 1994. When he came back home was when his disability started. Thank you God; I was able to catch up on the bills and get back on track. We had a nurse come in to take care of him while I was at work.

Those days were very hard for both of us and he knew it. He would sleep during the day and be up all night. We were in different bedrooms; he did not want to disturb me knowing I had to get up and go to work, because he would be in a lot of pain. He could not stand any covers on him, wearing shoes caused his feet to hurt, and he could not sit up long. He had a pillow to sit on that had a split in it so his tailbone could go into it, he had to sit on that pillow everywhere he went, even in the car.

People were talking about us, wanting to know what was wrong with us. He did not want anyone to know why he was dying. The only people that knew the truth were his mother and sister. We told everyone else that he had liver cancer. He did have jaundice but it was AIDS related.

Darryl moved back home with his mother one week before he died, so that he would have around the clock care. He called me at work on Friday October 14, 1994 to tell me he wanted to come back home. I told him I would pick him up after work. It was payday for me at the State Building, so I went out at lunch to cash my check and I got a corn beef sandwich for us to eat later when we got home. I knew I would not have time to cook or go grocery shopping.

As time progressed, Darryl had the death rattle in his voice. The nurse was not there yet, so he put my niece and nephews on the phone. I asked them where the nurse was, and they said she was on her way and was running late. Before I went to lunch, I talked to the nurse. She said he was slumped over in the bed and was having a hard time breathing, but not to worry she would get him stable. When I came back from lunch, I had an urgent message on my desk to call his mother's house. When I called, the nurse told me that the ambulance was taking him to South Point hospital and for me to get there as soon as I could.

I told my boss I needed to leave and I headed out the door. I did not have any gas in my car. I was riding on empty, but I got on the freeway downtown; by God's grace and mercy, I did not run out of gas. When I made it to South Point emergency room, my mother, his mother and sister were there in the waiting room waiting on me. I went back to see him and all he kept saying was he wanted to come home. I told him I would take him home after the doctors were finished checking him out and he was better. He started to take a turn for the worse. The doctors asked me if I wanted him to be resuscitated. I knew he had signed 'do not resuscitate' papers at University Hospital with Dr. Hutt, but we were at South Point; it did not matter what papers he signed at University Hospital.

Even though I knew he did not want to be, I still could not make that decision. I heard Darryl screaming my name so loud, I told the doctors to ask him. He sternly told the doctors that he had already signed papers and he did not want to be resuscitated; he just wanted to go in peace. They told him since he was at a different hospital than where he had signed those papers; they needed to know what his wishes were. I was so glad he could tell them himself.

They called University Hospital for Dr. Hutt, because they wanted to life flight him to where Dr. Hutt was; he asked them to put me on the phone. Dr. Hutt told me to look at a spot on the wall and I did. He told me not to allow them to life flight Darryl to University Hospital because there was nothing he could do for him. He said that Darryl was not going to make it and that he was already close to the other side. At this point, he said it would be best for them to give him some pain medicine to keep him pain free and comfortable. Dr. Hutt asked me was there anything I needed; I said no, my mother was with me to help me. She helped me stay focused on what I had to do and she kept my in-laws out of my way so I could make the decision I had to make as Darryl's wife.

They put Darryl in a room on Friday, October 14, 1994; his mother, sister and I stayed the night. My mother-in-law asked me to go home and change clothes first then come back and release her and my sister-in-law. I called my sister on my cell phone to come and get me from South Point, since my car did not have any gas. I left it in the hospital emergency parking lot. I knew Darryl had all his belongings including the truck at his mother's house. I had my sister take me over there, and the kids helped me load up the truck with all of Darryl's things. I knew when he died whatever items at his mother's house, I would not be able to get, so I made sure I got everything before I left. Due to an accident, the back door was rattling and dented; Darryl was trying to tell me about it at the hospital, but I did not know what he was saying.

I got home, took a hot bath, laid in the tub and let the phone ring; I needed time to myself. After a couple of hours I went to my mother's house, told her what I did and about the truck. She said, "The truck has insurance, your husband is dying. Get back to the hospital and worry about the truck later." I called my sister and she came and took me back to South Point. My mother-in-law and sister-in-law left to go home to change clothes.

Darryl was relaxing and talking. They had told me he would not even make it through Friday night and here it is Saturday, October 15, 1994. Darryl and I talked, he said he loved me and I said I loved him. He wanted something to eat; I called for him to get a tray and he ate it all. The nurse did not understand how he could eat, when all his organs were shutting down. He did ok with eating and it stayed down. When my mother-in-law and sister-in-law came back, I could see on my mother-in-law's face that she was not happy that I had been over to her house and got all Darryl's things and the truck, but she did not say a word.

Before Darryl went into the hospital he, told me to go and get the poem *Footprints in the Sand* off the shelf, that was what my niece and nephews had given him for a gift. I went to get it and brought it to Darryl. He said he finally understood the poem. I said, "You do? What does it mean?" He said, "God is carrying me. That's why it's only one set of footprints." I knew then that God was carrying Darryl. He had many talks with God. I knew then that Darryl's soul was saved and that he was safe in the arms of God. Darryl knew his life on this earth was ending. He did not want to live not being able to take care of himself, to work, play basketball, ride his motorcycle, be healthy and enjoy his life with his family.

Darryl was angry and hurt that his life was ending so soon. He asked many times, why did this have to happen to him. He said he was not strong enough to live with HIV/AIDS, but he told me he knew that I could and that I would. I did not think so, but

God had shown Darryl during all those talks and prayers he had with God.

Darryl asked me one day when I was lying on his chest in bed, if I could go on with my life or live in our house if he had died in it. He wanted to make sure I would be all right. Then all of a sudden, Darryl asked me was there anything I wanted to tell God, because God was in the room with us. I looked around and said, "Yes, I would."

"Well tell God he is here." He replied.

"God please help me stay strong and help me get through whatever I have to go through."

"God said He will and that He also will give you a whole, whole, whole lot more."

Then Darryl laughed and said, "She just don't know do she God?"

"Is it necessary to say, "Whole, whole lots that many times?"

Darryl laughed again and said, "Yes that many whole, whole, whole lots.

I could feel the presence of God in the room, but Darryl said he could see God. I truly believe God shown Darryl all he needed to see, to give him peace of mind. God let him know that he was with him every step of the way. We both said, "Thank you God."

Darryl's health went further downhill and his mother told him it was ok to let go. I went out in the hall and sat in a big recliner chair by the elevator doors; a big clock was hanging over the elevator. At 2:00 a.m. Sunday morning October 16, 1994, Darryl took his last breath. I saw doctors and nurses running saying code blue. I knew he was gone. I heard my in-laws crying and I let them stay in the room. I heard someone say, "Where is Kim?" They said I was in the hallway sitting in a chair. I went in by myself after my in-laws were done. I wanted to look Darryl over from head to toe, because he told me if he had any lesions on him, not to have an open casket. He did not want people to view him and see the lesions that were on him.

I would never forget the pain in Darryl's eyes. All he wanted was to be happy and have kids. Darryl wondered why his life had to end at a short time, but he also gave his life to Christ before he passed away.

## BEING POSITIVE

I tell you God is so good; every lesion on Darryl's body was gone. I could not believe it. I saw it with my own eyes. I had an open casket and Darryl looked like himself. His skin was smooth and he looked like he was just asleep. He looked like the handsome man I fell in love with and married; he was at peace. Thanks be to God.

*Kimberlin Dennis*
# BEING POSITIVE

## Chapter Five

After Darryl died, I did not care who knew I was infected with the disease. I could not keep the secret in any longer. People were talking about me everywhere: at home, in church, in the hospital, at work. This was coming from family, friends...everyone.

I was in the hospital after Darryl passed with pancreatitis and my T-cells were down to one and viral load was up to 19,000. My parents and doctor thought I was not going to make it, so they told my immediate family; they did not want me to die and my family not know why. I had people saying I was on drugs, or my husband was gay, or we were sexually active, none of it was true.

## BEING POSITIVE

I was mad at my parents for disclosing my status; no one asked me if I wanted people to know. Before I knew it I saw people from everywhere at my bedside. I knew that someone had to have said something; then my parents told me someone had. Well it was out, so I had to deal with it and I did not want to talk or see anyone.

I moved back home after Darryl died; I stayed in the house too. I would go outside to sit on the porch and the neighbors would say unpleasant things about me. They would say it loud enough for me to hear it. I would just go back into the house, until my mother said, "Let them talk, don't run from them, go sit on the porch and ignore them." and I did. My mother would tell me to hold my head up and do not be ashamed of what I was living with, just stay stress free and be happy.

It took me a year before I was able to talk about it. I was in denial and even though my parents had told my family, I did not want to talk about it. If people would ask me, I would tell them the truth, but I would never just bring it up to talk about. I wanted to keep the secret as long as I could, but God said no. I had to give a testimony. That was the first time I spoke out and told my story.

God was getting me ready to go out and speak, and start the Ministry of Hope. People still keep this secret to this day for the very same reasons I talked about. It is sad that 23 years later and people still feel like they cannot tell anyone.

*Kimberlin Dennis*
# BEING POSITIVE

## Chapter Six

When Dr. Hutt gave the news that I was HIV Positive, Darryl told Dr. Hutt not to worry about him, but just take care of his wife. Dr. Hutt said he would take care of us both. Dr. Hutt is still my doctor today.

My T-cells have dropped as low as one and have come back up as high as 400. My viral load has been as high as 19,000 and now I am undetectable. My viral load is less than 50 when I get my blood work done every three months; but it does not mean I am cured. HIV affects my immune system, my red blood cells and white blood cells.

After Darryl died, I got sick; I was taking AZT medication at that time. I kept getting pancreatitis and my T Cells were going down, down, down. The medication I was on seemed not to help. They had just come out with more medications because AZT was not working by itself, it needed help. They came out with a combination of pills. The regimen I was on at that time made me sick, but I kept praying, asking God what to do. My parents and sister did not want me to take the pills. It was all new to the doctors, as well as to the world. God said keep taking it.

I went through many different pills until Dr. Hutt found the right ones for me. The side effects from the pills are less but still can cause kidney problems. The pills were very big. I had one the size of a quarter. I had to crush it up and put it in something to drink to get it down. I was taking many pills; I think it was 32 pills a day. Now, I take 14 pills a day, seven in the morning from 6:30 a.m. - 7:00 a.m., and seven more from 6:30 p.m. - 7:00 p.m. One of my HIV medications, Viracept, has to be taken 12 hours apart; therefore, I take all my medications 12 hours apart.

I have to go see Dr. Hutt every three to four months. I get my blood taken to see where my T-cell and viral load counts are. Your T-cells are supposed to be high, a normal person has 600 to 1200 or higher, your viral load count is supposed to be low, zero/non-detectable. For some reason my T-cell count is between 200 to 400 or a little lower than 200, like 190. I do not know what a normal percentage is, but he said mine is good and it stays the same even if my T-cells fluctuates. My viral load is non-detectable, but understand that a person who has HIV/AIDS and has a non-detectable viral load still has the virus and is not cured. When

I get my blood taken, if the viral load is less than 50, then I am non-detectable. That is good; at one time, I had a viral load of 19,000 and 1 T-cell. Now I am non-detectable and my T cell count is 286.

Sometimes I miss a dose of medication, because I forget. It is not until I refill my pill case for the week that I realize I forgot to take the pills. Usually when I forget I only miss one dose not the whole day. For the most part, I try not to miss at all. My body can tell if I miss a dose, because I start feeling symptoms.

In the beginning, it was hard for me to take pills. I would get depressed about all the pills I had to take and I did not want to take them in front of people. They would say, "Girl why are you taking so many pills, and for what?" I did not want to tell people why I had to take them. The pills would make me sick and they left a nasty after-taste in my mouth. Now they have a coating on them so you do not smell or taste them going down. The smell and taste would make me sick, so I would hurry up and eat or drink something afterwards.

The medication started helping me, and my father said he was glad I listened to God and not my family. I knew they wanted what was best for me, and they felt like I was being treated as a guinea pig. I was, because the doctors did not know what the outcome would be. People were dying so fast back then, they really did not expect us to live this long. It is because of the medications, clinical trials, and research that we are now long-term survivors.

## BEING POSITIVE

I wish Darryl was still here, but he is not. I think about it all the time. A couple of times I wanted to give up, but God would send someone or something to me to remind me to not give up or throw in the towel, and to keep running the race. It is not about me, it is all about God. God uses me to educate and speak to his people. In a way I know it is not me talking; God comes in and takes control and its God talking. I feel the transformation God said, "Just trust me." and I do trust God. I did not think that I could or would be speaking and educating, I know it is a calling on my life. God knows just what I need, and he shows up right on time, all the time.

I continually pray and ask God to move me out the way and I ask Him to have His way. God said if I show up, He will show out.

## BEING POSITIVE

God has chosen people He wants me to bless. If I choose not to do the will of God, that is telling God no. My purpose is to be pleasing to God and God only. In doing so, God uses me to be a blessing to others.

My parents took care of me for three years when I was sick and then God said, "It's time to go." I looked for an apartment and I knew it had to be a place where God said so; where I could feel the presence of God in the place. When I called the number, I knew just talking on the phone it was the one. My cousin and I went to see the place. She ran a day care and she brought the kids with her. I felt God in the place and so did they. The kids were praising God in the living room and I was praising God in the bedroom. The apartment was being remodeled and it was going to take three to four months to finish. I was living with my parents, so I could wait.

The devil tried to trick me. The property owner said the apartment next door was done and if I wanted to, I could move in on my birthday, May 1st. In addition, it would only be 25 dollars more a month. I said I would let him know. I did not feel the presence of God in that one; it was at the back of the building and the one I felt God in was on the side of the building. I went back home to my parents' house, prayed to God on what to do. I did not want to make the wrong decision. God said, "Wait." I said, "God block it if it's not your will for me." and He did.

When I called the property owner the next day, before I could talk he said the apartment had been rented. A couple was coming from out of town, they were doctors, husband and wife, and they needed it right away. I told him good because I was calling to tell him I was going to wait on the one God wanted me to have. On July 1, 2000, I moved into my apartment and here it is 2017 and I am still in the same one.

God is good to me, to me, to me. My mother and some of my cousins were afraid of me moving out on my own. I prayed to God for me to be able to take care of myself. To eat, stay well, and not be dependent on my parents. My father and sister were all right with it but my mother, it took her some time. She had to see if I would be able to take care of myself.

I thank God that I had my parents' home to go back to, but I wanted my own place and space. I do not care how old I get; the rules are still the same at home with my parents. I have to pay rent, clean up, help around the house, and shut it down at a certain time of the night. I could have company, but not like, I wanted to. It is not as if it was my own place.

I have to eat right, exercise, and stay stress free. That is a daily routine for me and it works. I did not like to cook, I prayed for God to show me how to take care of myself and cook healthy meals to eat and I do. God promised me He would supply all my needs according to His riches and glory in Christ Jesus who strengthens me, and God does just that. Thank you God.

Dr. Hutt told me about the AIDS Task Force of Greater Cleveland. I went to my first women's support group, and I tell you 23 years later I am still going. Why? Because it helps me and I am there to help others. We help one another and I thank God for all the support groups at University Hospital, Metro Hospital, and Cleveland Clinic.

I put God first, read my bible every day, go to bible study and sing in the choir. I have belonged to Imani Church for 23 years now. I was going there before Darryl died and I joined a week later. I went back to New Light Baptist Church where I was baptized and grew up. My uncle was the pastor at the time. I could not talk about HIV/AIDS or even hear and learn God's word because everyone in our family was married or buried at New Light Church. I would only see funerals and weddings when I visited; but God sent me back there and I would go on Sundays, until licensed as a minister at Imani Church on January 15, 2016.

When I did not have to sing at Imani, I would go to the 8:00 a.m. service only and then I would go to New Light's 11:00 a.m. service. Imani has three services, 8:00 a.m., 10:00 a.m. and noon. Now, as a licensed minister, I attend all three services at Imani. I attend bible study on Tuesdays and choir rehearsal on Thursdays. My work on the Ryan White committee keeps me away from bible study on Wednesdays. I speak in schools and in the community; all of that is my support.

I do take time out to rest. When my body says rest, I listen and do so. If I cannot make it, it is ok. There have been times when I did not listen and God put me flat on my back where I had no other choice but to rest.

We videotaped all of the Christmas Holidays; from the time, my sister's kids were little. The kids would always enjoy looking at them from years past. On Christmas 2009, my mother had a cold and she was trying to stay away from me, because she knew my immune system was low. I caught a cold anyway, but it went from a cold to pneumonia.

I went into the hospital on January 18, 2009 with pneumonia. My mother would always take me to the doctor, but since she was sick, my father took me. We waited a long time for me to get a room; my father left and told me to call when they put me into one. It was about a six to eight hour wait for a room. It was full at the hospital; many people were sick.

I called my mother when I got into a room, it was after midnight and my mother was not happy that my father had left. She would have stayed with me until I got into a room, no matter how long it took. She worried about me all night. I told her to get well and I was going to get well also.

The next day my sister came to see me. We watched President Barack Obama be sworn in as the first black President of the United States of America. My sister and I were crying as we watched it on TV at my bedside in the hospital. Our mother called and she asked if we were watching it and my mother was crying as well. To see history for the first time, a black president in office. My mother told me to get well; she wanted to see me because she had not seen me since Christmas. We talked on the phone, but we did not see each other.

My third day in the hospital was Darryl's birthday, January 21. He would have been fifty years old then. My mother knew it was Darryl's birthday and she was worried about me in the hospital. I was worried about her because it had been since Christmas and she was still sick with a cold. We talked on the phone until 3:00 p.m., we told each other, "Love you, see you soon and get well."

Dr. Hutt came into the room to examine me. He said he had good news. The albuterol treatment was working, my breathing was getting better and that I could go home tomorrow. He said I could take a pill for the pneumonia when I got home. I was so happy I called my mother, but she did not answer the phone. I knew my father had to work at the Cavalier's game. He worked there just to have something to do after he retired from Ford Motor Co. He worked that night; it was a Wednesday. My parents also went to the store to buy food on Wednesdays. That was their shopping day. I thought maybe my father did not have to work and they went shopping instead. Worried I called my sister and she thought the same. I kept calling but no answer and it was getting late in the day. It was 11:00 p.m. and still no answer.

My friend came to see me. He bought me some chicken to eat and we played cards to keep my mind off it, but I knew something was not right. I called my sister's house again, all I could hear was my sister crying and screaming that mama is dead. My nephew answered the phone and he said, "Grandma is dead." I told the nurse to call Dr. Hutt and tell him to let me go home now; I could not wait until morning. She did and Dr. Hutt released me. I signed the papers so I could go home. Dr. Hutt said I had to promise him that I would take care of myself when I went home.

It was so cold outside and snowing hard. You could not see in front of you. I called my best girlfriend and told her. She had her husband bring her to the hospital where I was. I was far out on Som Center Road and it is far from my house, about 20 minutes away on a good day. You have to get on the freeway to get there. My girlfriend and her husband pulled up just as my friend and I were leaving. I had him take me to my parents' apartment, which is across the street from where I live. I knew I could not go back and forth, due to the cold weather.

My father did not know that I knew my mother was dead. He did not want me to know, due to my health. When I walked in, my father was in shock. He asked, "How did you find out?" I said, "I called my sister's house and I heard her screaming mama is dead, so I had Dr. Hutt release me from the hospital because I could not stay there overnight." I went and got into my parents' bed and cried my eyes out.

I stayed with my father until after the funeral. My mother had a heart attack and my father found her on the living room floor when he came home from working the Cavaliers game. I helped get my mother ready for the viewing. Her hairdresser did her hair and I was glad because my mother would have wanted her own hairdresser to fix her up. He did and my mother's hair was beautiful. I had to do my oldest sister's, great grandmother's and grandmother's hair when they died. I would have done my mother's too if I had to. I was there when her hairdresser did it. I only went outside when I had to, but I did not stay long; just to do what needed to be done. I had to remember that I was sick and it was still cold out and snowing. I took my medication and did everything I promised Dr. Hutt I would do to stay well.

After that was over, in November 2009, I was in the bathroom brushing my teeth and I felt a lump in my left breast. I thought it was another duct leak, because back in 2001 this same breast had a duct leak in it. I had surgery to plug it up; it was fine until 2009 when I felt the lump. I called the same doctor who did the surgery before. He had me come in and scheduled me for surgery again. This was in December of 2009 after Christmas.

On January 5, 2010, I received a call from the doctor telling me to come in to discuss the next step because I was diagnosed with stage two-breast cancer. My father went with me. The doctor told me I had to start chemotherapy and radiation right away. I pray about everything and I had already prayed to God on how to handle this. I did the same thing when I was diagnosed with HIV/AIDS, and God enabled me to be a fifteen-year survivor. I told the doctor no chemo, but he wanted to start me on it as soon as possible. I told my father, "Let's go."

I came home, called Dr. Hutt, and told him what I was going through. Dr. Hutt had me come to his office. He asked me what I wanted to do. I said I wanted a second opinion. Dr. Hutt said, "I have a doctor for you and this is a doctor I would recommend my wife to if she were in your shoes." I love Dr. Hutt. I went to this new doctor, had a second surgery and they took nine lymph nodes out and two were cancerous. The MRI, CT SCAN, and Mammogram did not show the cancer. I could feel the lump and so could the doctor. I do not know why it did not show up on the test.

After the second surgery, my doctor told me I did not have to have chemo, but I did have to have six and a half weeks of radiation and I did. Eight years later and my health is well. It was good I did not do chemo, it would have taken all the T-cells I had, and I do not have many as it is. My doctor said we made the right decision, but I know it was God. I thank God for my being obedient to him and him only. God is good to me, to me, to me.

## Chapter Seven

After being diagnosed for a year, my husband was gone and I moved back home to live with my parents. During this time, God began to get my attention. I spent a lot of time praying and crying. At one point, I did not eat for an entire week. My father told me I needed to eat or I would get sick and cause my health to get worse. Unconsciously God had me fasting for the first time in my life.

I started going to church at Imani before Darryl died. I told him that I had been visiting but he did not have a chance to attend before he died. Every Sunday, I ran home to repeat the message to Darryl. I did not want him to miss the empowering word of God that was getting me through each day. After Darryl died, I joined Imani church the following week.

I needed to be surrounded by positivity as much as possible.

It took a long time for me to accept my diagnosis; initially I did not tell anyone that I was HIV Positive. I thought I only needed to attend Sunday morning services, until I went to a conference for the first time. The first night of the conference was on a Friday. There was a guest speaker by the name Rae Lewis-Thornton, 'Diva Living with AIDS'. I did not know her; she was the first black woman on Oprah's show, who told her story living HIV positive. I watched her tell her story and as she was talking, I was sitting in the back crying my eyes out. I said to myself, "How can she do that?" God showed me through her what He wanted me to do. In my mind's eye, I could see God taking her out of her shoes and put me in them. I could see me walking up and down the sanctuary, telling my story living with HIV/AIDS.

I did not tell a soul. I went home, went to sleep, and had a dream. God said, "I'm the Ministry of Hope." I wondered what he meant by saying, "I'm the Ministry of Hope." I woke up and all that came out of my mouth was "Ministry of Hope." My mother was in the kitchen cooking. I sat and watched her cook, she was talking to me and all that would come out of my mouth was, "Ministry of Hope." My mother kept asking me why I was not answering her and saying, "Ministry of Hope." I called my cousin Jackie and she said, "God wants you to start the Ministry of Hope."

The Ministry of Hope was born and I began telling my story. I began speaking in colleges, churches, schools, prerelease centers, jails, wherever God would send me; and I will continue to go wherever He leads me. My best friend Linda, from elementary school and all through middle and high school, gave me the name, "Girl on a Mission". Every time she would call, I would be doing a program or speaking somewhere and she would tell people, "That's my girl on a mission." Girl on a mission is about doing the will of God, no matter what it takes.

Once I was speaking on HIV/AIDS and while I was sharing my story, I found myself getting off track talking about my sister Robin's murder. I kept trying to get back on track. The Holy Spirit would not let me. This was the first time I had ever experienced this situation during a speaking engagement. I kept fighting with myself about getting back on track, but after I finished my speech, someone in the class shared their experience were their sister had been murdered the same way. This person thought they were the only one who had experienced a tragedy like that in their family. At that moment, I knew that it was God's will for me to share my experience of my sister's murder.

From that day forward, I do not worry about getting off track. Every time it happens, it is for a reason. So many pieces of my testimony has help others. Outside of the HIV infection, I have gained strength through every other obstacle of my life.

Another time I was speaking and telling my story when a person asked me how I could come in and speak like I did in front of people.

I said, "It's the will of God." God called me to speak, I did not want to, nor did I think I was capable to speak. This person said they had something that they wanted to say. I opened the floor so they could have a chance to speak.

One of the individuals shared the details of her experience of being raped. The person who raped them lived in the building where we were. She was afraid it would happen again so she took the police and showed them where the assailant lived. She felt she deserved the attack because of her location.

I explained to her that no one deserves to be raped. I talked to everyone there that heard the story and informed everyone not to tell anyone outside that place. I told them to support this woman and explained that she was not the only one who has experienced this tragedy.

This individual was brave enough to say something and do something about it, like take the police over to that person's house, identify that person, and make a report on it. I told this person that they needed to get professional counseling. I also said, "Do not blame yourself, you did the right thing." I reminded everyone they had the right to say no; no one should be violated no matter what location they were in or who they are.

A one-hour speaking engagement turned into a three-hour session. I had to make sure that the people who heard it was not going to let it out of the room, and I had to make sure they were there to support this person and not discriminate against them. I was not expecting something like that to happen, but I prayed and asked God to come in and take over to help me help this person in the right way and God did. He used me to not only help this individual, but also every person that was in the room that day. I could not leave until I felt the peace of God and knowing that I did all I could to help this person.

A month or two later I was watching the news and I saw that they had caught the person who had done this. That day I cried and thanked God for using me to help this person to stand strong and do the right thing for themselves and others. If that person did it once, they could have done it again to someone else. I thank God for the victory. As I said, many times, I went to educate and speak on

HIV/AIDS; I got off track and found myself in a different situation.

There was a time I was helping another person who was HIV positive; he did not want to live. He was doing drugs and wanted to die. He was not taking care of himself. I was trying to encourage him to want to live again. Reassuring him that HIV/AIDS was not a death sentence and he could live a long life if he chose to.

Life is about the choices we make. I choose to live, so I do whatever I need to do to take care of myself: eat right, exercise and stay stress free. When people find out that they are HIV positive, they lose hope and do not want to live. Some turn to drugs or drinking and they do not take care of their health. When a person is doing drugs, they do not care whom they have sex with or what type of sex it is. The person I was trying to help did not care, and did not inform people of their HIV status before having sex. I asked them how they could do this. They were angry about being infected and only wanted the drugs. Personally, I would have told the other person I am HIV positive. I told them that it was the right thing to do and eventually they told their sex/drug partner they were HIV positive. Not long after that, he died. The HIV did not kill this person; the drugs did.

I used to worry about dying with HIV/AIDS, now I just live my life to the fullest. My life could have ended in other ways besides HIV/AIDS. I do not worry now as I used to in the beginning. People were dying so fast back when I was diagnosed and my husband was one of them. No one thought people with HIV/AIDS could live long. Now we are long time survivors.

Over the years of teaching and speaking on HIV/AIDS, I took the class and became a certified tester. I always wondered what I would do if someone came up positive during one of my programs or events. The first time it happened, my first positive, it was an indescribable feeling. Why, because I knew the pain, hurt, and denial I felt and now someone else was walking in my shoes. I prayed for this person, but I did not know at that time who the person was. I was doing the education that day, and someone else from the health department did the testing for me.

A week went by and the person came to a function where I was. They started crying so hard they had to be taken out the room. There were about three other people helping this person. When I showed up this person screamed they were HIV positive. I had to lock the room we were in, tell the other people to keep what was said in the room, and then help the person who was positive get them self together. I told them where to go to get treatment and help, where to go for support and who to talk with. I talked to this person and shared all I could. I wanted to make sure this person was not trying to give up on life. God is so good. He gave me the right words to say. I helped this person today and this individual is doing well, taking care of them self and living a good life. Thanks be to God.

A large part of my journey is going to support groups and I encourage others to go to one too. They help me and I see how they also help others. It is important for me to see the doctor, get regular checkups and take my medication to stay on top of any problem that may occur. I find myself in many missions. God is truly using me for His glory. My purpose is to stop the spread of HIV/AIDS, and to help as many people as I can. Just knowing I am making a positive impact in the world is a blessing.

The bible says if I get to one, my job is done. I thank God for the many. God is good to me, to me, to me. All of the missions God sends me on are more good than bad. I have numerous stories to tell that are good.

One of them is when I was out shopping on Black Friday and I was in a HH Gregg store looking around. I went over to look at the mattresses, lie on them and price them so I would already know the one I wanted when I got ready to buy one. A salesperson saw me lying on the mattress, he said, "Miss Dennis, is that you?" I said, "Yes," and he said, "Do you remember me?" I said, "No, where should I remember you from?" He explained that I came to speak at his school when he was in the eighth grade. I remembered going to his school, and he said he was home from college and was working at HH Gregg for the holidays. The young man thanked me. He said I helped change his life for the better. It is because of me coming to his school and telling my story, that he is a good person now. He hugged me and thanked me. I told him good, keep up the good work. He said that he will never forget me, and he told all his friends about me.

## BEING POSITIVE

You see, God is so good. I remembered he was one of the kids that was giving me a hard time in the class that day. Sometimes I think the kids are acting up or lashing out, because they do not want to pay attention. I did not know what his reason was that day, but I thank God that he did learn something. I tell the kids all the time, especially the ones that are disrespectful, that I hope they never have to walk in my shoes. I hope no one ever gets HIV/AIDS. That is why I do what I do.

One time I was going to the store to get a birthday gift for my great nephew and niece. Their birthdays are three days apart. They were having a birthday party at Fun 'n' Stuff. I did not want to go unless I had a gift for them. This was March of 2013. I went to JC Penney, Macy's, Sears, Target and I could not find anything. I came all the way home, took off my coat, lay across my bed, and I heard the Holy Spirit say get up and go to Wal-Mart. I looked around the room and said, "Yeah, right. I have been to four stores and could not find what I wanted. Now God, you say 'get up and go to Wal-Mart.'" I got up and went to Wal-Mart on Richmond Road where the Holy Spirit said to go. I walked in and saw the outfits for the kids, as if they were waiting for me. I could not believe it. I got them and went to the checkout line to pay for them.

A woman pulled up behind me in a wheelchair cart. She was talking on her cell phone. When I turned back around she had left the cart there and walked away talking on her phone; the cart was full of items. I had two people in line in front of me and the line kept moving up. A woman passed by with three girls and asked me was someone in line behind me. I said, "Yes, but she walked away, talking on her cell phone." At that time, the three girls told their mother that they knew me. She did not believe them and went to the next line to check out.

Before I could check out, the woman walked over to me in a different demeanor. She explained that although she did not know how her daughters knew me she knew there was something I said to them that changed their lives drastically. I did not know exactly what to do, but I prayed that God would guide me. She thanked me for saving her daughters' lives. She explained that she was not sure what I said to them, but she wanted to show her gratitude for the impact that I had on their lives.

At that moment, God said it was ok for me to share with her on what I do in the schools as a person living with HIV/AIDS. The mother said her girls were sexually active and were out in the streets. Nothing she did or said had stop them, but when they met me and heard my story at their school, it changed their lives for the better. Since then she has not had any trouble out of them. They do not give up their bodies for sex anymore and choose to stay abstinent. I said, "Thank you God."

I knew then that was why I could not find anything in the other four stores. God sent me to Wal-Mart to receive the blessing from that mother and her three girls. I was trying to stop speaking. I was ready to throw in the towel. However, God said no, and to look at the many people who were blessed because I go out and do what thus said the Lord. Therefore, you see the good always outweighs the bad. I have to continue to look at the bigger picture as my mother told me a long time ago.

When I first started to speak, I would have kids that were so rude; it would have me in tears. I would call my mother crying, she would say it is ok, do not give up and to look at the bigger picture. There are more being blessed than the one or two who were not listening.

*Kimberlin Dennis*
# BEING POSITIVE

## Chapter Eight

Being an African American, straight woman, we are the number one infected with HIV/AIDS. All African Americans are number one in infection. The disease does not discriminate; it has no race, age, color, or face. You are either infected with HIV/AIDS or you are affected by it. It is not easy to be in a relationship with someone who is not infected. Not to say there are no such relationships, but there are more positive women who want to be in a relationship with a negative man but are not. The virus we live with stigmatizes us.

After I gave a testimony at Imani church, God was preparing me for the Ministry of Hope. I started giving programs at the church trying to educate as many people as possible. I knew I had to tell my story. My husband did not want anyone in his family or

117

friends to know, only his mother and sister knew the truth. I had Dr. Hutt tell Darryl my results two weeks after his in front of both of them; he had a doctor's appointment at the same time I got my results. Darryl said he was not strong enough to deal with people knowing, but when he passed, God said it is time. Darryl told me that he knew I would be strong and live with HIV so when I speak, I tell our story and I say, "Darryl, we have to help one more person if not many to help stop the spread of HIV/AIDS."

I step out on faith and trust God. God promised me He would never leave me, nor forsake me. God promised me He would be with me every step of the way. I do not write down what I want to say, I speak from my heart and God always shows up and shows out every time. God is good to me, to me, to me. Speaking helps me to stay stress free. I talk about the good, the bad and the ugly. People can relate when you are real and they know you are speaking from your heart. They can feel it. I see the transformation from the time I say I am HIV positive to the end of my speaking. I chose to stay abstinent until marriage, so I stress the importance of abstinence. It is not easy, but with God, all things are possible.

I used to count at the end of the year how many people I have reached, but the number has gotten so big now I just say billions of people. I still count how many at each speaking or program and keep a record but it is just a habit. The largest speaking engagement was at Hampton College in

Hampton, VA with about 600 people in one room.

## Chapter Nine

When Darryl died, I was afraid to be in a relationship. I had an old boyfriend; we dated when I was in junior high. We had never had sex but this man was in love with me. He was older than I was, so I broke up with him to date someone my age that was in the same school as me. The old boyfriend was also close to the family.

He came back to me after Darryl died and wanted to marry me. I said no because I could not tell him I was HIV positive and we were kids and that was puppy love to me. I told him I knew he loved me, I asked him to give me time to see if I could fall in love with him. We dated for a few months without having intercourse. I felt it was time to tell him my status. We went down to the 72$^{nd}$ street pier by the lake, we sat at a picnic table and I told him my status. I cried my eyes out and he told me he knew already. He heard about my status when my parents told the immediate family but he wanted me to tell him myself. I thought that was over and out the way and that he would be ok.

After we dated for a couple of years still there was no intercourse. I noticed he was not asking me to marry him and he was very distant. He was seeing this woman but he lied and said he was not. I caught him, but he still to this day denied it. We broke up because he felt we could not have sex and he wanted to have more kids. He already had two from a previous marriage.

My relationship with my family is good. Everyone in my family knows my status. I no longer get the rejection I did in the beginning. My relationship with my friends is good. My friends are mostly people in the spectrum living with HIV/AIDS like me. I have a few girlfriends that have been my friends from the very beginning. I never had many friends, but I can say four girlfriends have been with me before HIV/AIDS and still are today.

I have one best friend for life; he is also in the spectrum. We are just friends; I cannot see us married. We did not have intercourse, but when we met in 2005, we did have protected sexual relations. I got sick and ended up in University Hospital and God spoke to me and said STOP, so I did.

I have to practice what I preach. I am not in a relationship. I have friends that I go out with, spend time with, but we do not have sex. I am abstinent and I choose to stay that way until God gives me the right man for me and we get married.

Being HIV positive is so hard for women who want to date or have a relationship. We have to disclose our status and that is ok. We also do not want to go to jail for being in a relationship with someone, realize it is not working out and that person lies and says they did not know our status. They are mad at the fact that you both can no longer be together so they use your HIV/AIDS status against you.

It is sad that the world is like that. So many of us single, good women are alone today just because we have HIV/AIDS and no one wants us or we are afraid of getting caught up in a lawsuit. I stay abstinent because for me it is the right thing to do. When I go out to speak, I share with the people that I'm abstinent. I know how important it is to say no. I tell the kids it is ok to say no. It is not easy, but with God, all things are possible.

I would not be able to do this without God. I do not think about sex or even having it. I prayed for God to help me to live abstinent. It has been many years now and it probably will be many more. I know if God gives me a husband, I could have protected sex like Magic Johnson and his wife. Therefore, there is hope, but until then I do not think about it or even have the urge anymore.

*Kimberlin Dennis*
# BEING POSITIVE

## Chapter Ten

Today I am at peace. I go out, speak, and educate on HIV/AIDS as a person living with the disease. I have a nonprofit organization, Ministry of Hope; Inc. Speaking is a stress release for me. Just knowing I have reached one person, if not many, my job is complete. The after effect is so awesome, when years later, I see or hear about someone who met me or heard my story and it helped him or her to make good changes in life. They testify to me on how I helped them to be the person they are today.

It is hard for people who have HIV/AIDS to be in a relationship. Being an African American woman that is all you hear; we cannot get married because no one wants to be with us, because of our HIV status. When talking to someone, I see if this is someone I like, or who likes me. If I feel it could be someone I would like to continue talking to, then I will tell that person my status. If we are just friends and I know this is not the one for me or we are not doing any type of sexual acts, then no. Not everyone needs to know my status. Only if you are going to be in a relationship with that person, then it is best for that person to know before the relationship goes on.

Most of the time when we disclose our status, people say, "Oh no, never mind." We deal with rejection a lot and it hurts when you are rejected because of your HIV/AIDS status. That is why it is hard for us to be in a relationship in the first place. You see TV shows where people are getting a date and having a relationship with a good man, like the

Steve Harvey show. That is good, but people like myself ask, "What about people who are infected with HIV/AIDS? Is there someone for us?" Everyone wants a romantic partner or wants to be happy and have a good relationship. There are very few cases like that for people whom have HIV/AIDS. A woman will take a man that is living with HIV/AIDS, before a man will take a woman who is living with HIV/AIDS.

Being in a relationship with someone, you have to make sure that the person understands Ohio Law. The Ohio Law (Referred to as House Bill 100) says that if a person has HIV/AIDS and does not tell their partner before having sex (even if you are practicing safe sex), it is a crime or felony for anyone diagnosed with HIV or AIDS. Before any sexual act, you have to tell your partner your status and ask your partner to sign a paper stating that you told them you are infected with HIV/AIDS, or have someone you know and trust listen to you tell your sex partner that you are HIV positive. That person can be your witness. An HIV positive person who has sex without telling his or her partner about the HIV commits a second-degree felony. This means that if the person is convicted the sentence will be less than it would be for a first-degree felony like murder.

I do not want to give HIV/AIDS to anyone nor do I want to go to jail for being in a relationship with someone who ends up using my HIV status against me. Very few people are in a relationship who have HIV/AIDS for this very reason.

What are our options; should we just be alone for the rest of our lives or do we have the right to be happy and be in a relationship and get married someday? It seems like it is easy for two people who are positive to be in a relationship because you both know each other's status and know what each other is dealing with. I did not choose to be infected, but I have it, so does that mean I do not live life to the fullest? Why can't someone like myself be happy? Why can't I have a man who is not HIV positive that loves me for who I am just the way I am and we both be happy and live a life together?

Using condoms is a source of protection, but they are not 100% effective because they can break and let the virus in. If your T-cell count is good and your Viral Load is undetectable, then there is a very slim chance of infecting someone else. Because you are infected, people are afraid so they choose to abstain from any relationships. It is not good, but this is life.

I want people to know that there is hope. Why? Because they are getting closer to a cure, and to love yourself for who you are, just the way you are. God will give you peace of mind. We are not alone. Go to support groups to help yourself get through life, seek professional help from a psychiatrist, take good care of your body, take your medication, eat and stay stress free. We are all born to die, but it is what we do while we are living that counts. "I can do all things through Christ who gives me strength."

## BEING POSITIVE

Everyone has a story; let your story empower, inspire and encourage someone else to believe, to live and be happy. When people look at me or hear me speak I want them to know and say, "If Kimberlin Dennis can do it, so can I." To God be the glory! God is good to me, to me, to me. It is my voice, but it is God speaking through me. It is my presence, but it is God's Holy Spirit and power. It is my story, but its God's will for my life to be an inspiration to others. To help, to love, and to know we are strong.

*Kimberlin Dennis*
# BEING POSITIVE

24120975R00074

Made in the USA
Columbia, SC
20 August 2018